Table of Contents

When shopping at the grocery store, the foods you grab can greatly impact your overall health. In fact, filling your cart with a lot of refined grains, sugary drinks, and processed foods can increase inflammation and affect your health.

Therefore, filling up on healthy foods can help keep you healthy, protect against chronic diseases resistant to drugs and rid your body of toxins.

We also absorb tons of toxins every day through the air we breathe, the water we drink, the food we eat, and by just being outside in our surroundings.

So how do we get rid of these toxins that can be harmful to our body? It's through the Healing diet.

The Healing foods diet is not just a diet; It is a tool that will lead you to a total transformation of your health. This diet was designed to help everyone overcome diseases. It is designed to heal your body and improve your health by encouraging the consumption of nutritious, whole foods like fruits, veggies, legumes, healthy fats, organic meats, and healing herbs and spices.

Plus, this simple eating pattern is a great way to ensure you supply your body with a steady stream of the nutrients you need to help prevent nutritional deficiencies in your diet and to promote healthy living.

So what makes this diet unique?

This diet is unique because it involves making some simple switches in your diet compared to other complicated diets with many rules and regulations.

1. Turkey Meatloaf with Cranberry Apple Chutney

Prep: 25 mins

Cook: 1 hr

Total: 1 hr 25 mins

Servings: 6

Ingredients

For the Meatloaf:

- 2 lbs ground turkey
- 1 large carrot, shredded
- ¼ cup rolled oats
- ¼ cup oat milk
- 1 flax egg 1 tbsp ground flax + 3 tbsp cool water, set aside for 15 mins
- 1 tbsp dried parsley
- 1 tsp dried basil
- 1 tsp dried oregano

- ½ tsp garlic powder

- 1 tsp salt

- ½ tsp black pepper

For the Chutney:

- 3 green apples, peeled and shredded

- 1 yellow onion diced

- ¼ cup dried cranberries

- 1 tbsp white wine vinegar

- ¼ tsp turmeric

- 1 tsp ground ginger

- ½ tsp cumin

- 1 tsp salt

- olive oil

Directions

For the Meatloaf:

1. Preheat oven to 350 degrees F

2. mix all ingredients in a large bowl, shape into a loaf and place in a large greased baking pan.

3. Bake for 1 hour, at about the halfway point remove from oven and carefully drain the liquids from the pan (make sure internal temp reaches 160 degrees F)
4. Serve topped with chutney.

For the Chutney

1. Heat a medium pan over medium low heat, drizzle pan with olive oil.
2. Add onions and saute until they become soft.
3. Add the remaining ingredients and simmer until the apple juice is evaporated and the mixture just begins to become sticky, this may take a while but don't be tempted to turn the heat up too high.
4. Serve warm on top of meatloaf.

Prep: 10 mins

Cook: 1 hr 15 mins

Total: 1 hr 25 mins

Servings: 4

Ingredients

- 1 13.5 oz can full-fat canned coconut milk
- 1.5 tbsp pure maple or honey
- 1 tsp gelatin
- 1 tbsp chia seeds
- Zest 1 lemon
- 1-2 cups berries For topping later!
- Berry Topping
- 1 cup frozen raspberries (or any berries you have on hand!)
- 1.5 tbsp honey or pure maple
- Juice from one lemon

Directions

1. Open canned coconut milk and stir with a spoon until oil and cream are well mixed.

2. Remove ⅓ of the canned milk and pour in a pan. Heat until just boiling and divide into two small bowls.

3. In one bowl, sprinkle in the gelatin until it blooms (AKA starts to ripple and take shape.) After 3-4 min, whisk together until dissolved and slightly frothy.

4. In the other bowl, stir in sweetener and lemon zest.

5. Combine the two bowls of split coconut milk and then the remaining coconut milk from the can.

6. Lastly, add the chia and stir well until seeds are evenly dispersed. Refrigerate for at least 1 hr and 15 minutes. (You could always make the base the night before and the compote fresh the next morning for breakfast.)

Berry Topping:

1. Combine all ingredients in a saucepan on low to medium heat until water has evaporated and berries are soft and broken down.

2. Take fresh berries and dump evenly across four small glasses (6-10 oz). A few inches is great.

3. Divide entire batch of coconut cream across four glasses.

4. Top cream with warm berry topping and additional fresh berries.

5. Feel free to add additional crunch if you have it on hand such as cacao nibs, hemp seeds, flax, nuts, or elimination diet approved granola. Cover and refrigerate until ready to serve.

Prep: 5 mins

Refrigerate: 12 hrs

Total: 12 hrs 5 mins

Servings: 1

Ingredients

- ½ cup rolled oats
- 1 cup coconut milk
- ½ cup berries, mango, sliced peaches, whatever fruit you like
- 2 tbsp sweetened shredded coconut
- ¼ tsp cinnamon
- pinch salt

Directions

1. Add all ingredients to a sealable single serving container
2. Sit in fridge overnight and enjoy cold.

Prep: 15 mins

Cook: 8 mins

Total: 23 mins

Servings: 4

Ingredients

- 1 tbsp Vital Proteins Collagen Gelatin
- 3/4 cup coconut flour
- 1/2 cup cassava flour
- 1/2 cup coconut milk or any nut or seed milk of your choice.
- 3 tbsp hot water
- 3 tbsp 100% pure maple syrup
- 1-2 tsp cinnamon
- Coconut oil for cooking
- Toppings of choice for pancakes We love berries, warm nut butter and cacao nibs!

Directions

1. Add hot water to a small glass cup and sprinkle gelatin on top.

2. Combine both flours and cinnamon in a medium sized bowl.

3. Add the coconut milk, maple, gelatin mixture and whisk well. (Sometimes heating the milk before mixing can help to keep the mixture warm which makes for a smoother blending process.)

4. Heat your favorite non-toxic pan to medium low heat then add a spoonful of coconut until evenly melted. Take an ice cream scooper to scoop a few portions of batter across your pan.

5. Let it cook for 3-5 minutes then flip and cook for another 2-3 minutes.

6. Pancake should harden a bit in texture and turn slightly light brown. Set on plate and enjoy!

Tip: Top pancakes with whatever excites you most on your pancakes, almond butter and berries, 100% pure maple syrup, cacao nibs, hemp seeds etc.!

Prep: 10 mins

Cook: 15 mins

Total: 25 mins

Servings: 4

Ingredients

- 2/3 cup cassava flour
- 1/4 cup coconut flour
- 1 tsp baking soda
- 1/2 cup melted coconut oil
- 1/4 cup honey
- 1/4 cup unsweetened applesauce
- 1/2 cup dried unsweetened cranberries
- 2 tbsp orange zest
- 1/4 tsp salt

Directions

1. Preheat oven to 350 degrees and grease your favorite non-toxic cookie sheet.

2. In a medium bowl combine both flours, baking soda, orange zest and salt.

3. Gently stir until evenly mixed. Mix in honey, applesauce, and coconut oil until a well mixed thick batter is formed.

4. Fold in cranberries. Use an overflowing tablespoon to scoop out about 16 mounds of batter across your cookie sheet.

5. Bake for approximately 15 minutes or until firm and golden brown. Enjoy once completely cooled.

Prep: 30 mins

Cook: 20 mins

Total: 50 mins

Servings: 4

Ingredients

- 1 lb lean ground beef
- 1 yellow onion, diced
- 1 carrot shredded
- 8 oz white or baby bella mushrooms, sliced
- 3 cloves garlic, minced
- 2 medium sweet potatoes, large chopped
- 2 tbsp coconut oil or other neutral flavored oil
- ¼ cup oat milk or any plain milk
- 1 tsp dried rosemary
- 1 tsp oregano
- salt
- pepper

- olive oil

Directions

1. Preheat the oven to 350 degrees F
2. Brown the ground beef in a large skillet over medium heat.
3. Remove the beef to drain and set aside.
4. Saute the onion, carrot, and mushrooms in the beef fat for about 10 minutes until the mushrooms release their juices.
5. Meanwhile bring the sweet potatoes to a boil in a medium pot, start with cool water and bring it up to the boil for about 15 minutes until the sweet potatoes mash easily with a fork.
6. Add the minced garlic, rosemary, and oregano to the vegetables and saute an additional minute
7. Drain the potatoes and mash with a masher, fork, or mixer with the coconut oil and milk.
8. Stir the beef into the vegetable mix.
9. Lightly grease a 7X11 pan.

10. Put the beef and vegetable mix into the greased pan.

11. Scoop the sweet potatoes on top to form an even layer.

12. Bake for 20 minutes until the potatoes form a slight crust.

13. Serve hot.

Prep: 5 mins

Cook: 5 mins

Total: 10 mins

Servings: 2

Ingredients

- 1 large sweet potato
- Your choice of toppings

Hint: You can go sweet with options like peanut butter, banana and cinnamon or almond butter and cacao nibs or you can opt for savory like smashed avocado with sea salt and pepper or hummus, smoked salmon or even a fried egg!

Directions

1. Take the sweet potato and slice it lengthwise into approximately ¼ inch thick pieces.

2. Toast for 4-6 minutes in your toaster. (It may take a little longer for it to be cooked through depending on the power of your toaster.)

3. Top with desired toppings.

4. Place an extra slice on top if you are more of a sandwich fan or leave it open-faced like traditional toast. Either way, enjoy!

8. Cinnamon Banana Porridge

Prep: 8 hrs

Cook: 5 mins

Total: 8 hrs 5 mins

Servings: 4

Ingredients

- ½ cup almonds
- ½ cup walnuts or macadamia nuts
- 1 ripe banana
- 1 can of unsweetened coconut milk
- 1 overflowing spoonful of cashew butter or almond
- 2 tsp cinnamon

Directions

1. Soak nuts in water overnight then drain.

2. Use a blender or food processor to blend nuts, banana, canned coconut milk, cinamon and nut butter.

3. Pour into a small pan on stovetop and eat on low.

4. Divide batch in half and serve.

Prep: 15 mins

Cook: 15 mins

Total: 30 mins

Servings: 2

Ingredients

Steak:

- 1/2 lb grass-fed top sirloin, a bigger steak yields wonderful leftovers
- 4-5 garlic cloves, crushed or minced
- 1/4 cup extra virgin olive oil
- Nachos
- 1 cup cooked black beans, or 3/4 cup canned beans drained
- 1/2 cup salsa or 1 cup Pico de Gallo
- 1 cup tear drop tomatoes, cut in half
- 1 cup Simple Healthy Guacamole

- 30 Homemade Sweet Potato Chips, or Terra's Veggie Chips

Directions

For the Steak:

1. Place steak in a shallow glass pan.
2. Mince or crush garlic & spread over top of steak. Drizzle steak with olive oil.
3. Cover and marinate in refrigerator for 1-3 hours for first side. Once first side is marinated, remove garlic, flip steak and cover second side with original garlic.
4. Cover and marinate again in refrigerator for 1-3 hours. 1 hour before grilling, remove from refrigerator and let the steak come up to room temperature.
5. Heat grill over a medium/high heat, making sure grill is fully heated before using.
6. Place steak on grill and do not touch until you see a small amount of blood rise to the surface. Flip steak, refrain from touching again until a small

amount of blood rises to the surface again. Cooking times will be approximately 7 mins per side.

7. Once grilled, remove from heat and let rest for about 10 mins.

8. Add salt & pepper to taste. Then slice against the grain in medium sized stripes and then into chunks for the nachos.

For the Nachos:

1. Heat beans in a medium sauce pan over medium/low heat or in glass saucepan with lid in the microwave for 8 minutes on power level 8.

2. Divide Homemade Sweet Potato chips between 2 plates and top with beans, tomatoes, salsa, steak and guacamole.

Prep: 5 mins

Servings: 1

- 1 cup frozen, fresh, or canned peach slices (loosely packed)
- ½ cup vanilla coconut yogurt
- ½ cup coconut milk
- 2 tbsp honey or real maple syrup
- ½ tsp vanilla extract
- pinch salt

Directions

1. Blend all ingredients in a food processor or blender until smooth
2. Serve cold

Prep: 20 mins

Cook: 4 hrs

Total: 4 hrs 20 mins

Servings: 5

Ingredients

- 6 chicken thighs boneless/skinless or bone in with skin removed
- 1 yellow onion chopped
- 2 large carrots chopped large
- 1 stalk celery diced
- 3 cloves garlic minced
- 1 ½ cups chicken broth
- 2 tbsp apple cider vinegar
- 2 tsp ground cumin
- ½ tsp cinnamon
- 1 tsp ground ginger
- ½ tsp coriander

- ¼ tsp ground turmeric
- 2-3 tsp salt or to taste
- ¼ tsp black pepper
- 1 tbsp olive oil
- ⅓ cup green olives
- ⅓ cup golden raisins
- 3 cups cooked basmati rice

Directions

1. Place chicken thighs in slow cooker and drizzle lightly with olive oil.
2. Add all other ingredients except the olives, raisins, and cooked rice.
3. Cook on high for 4 hours.
4. If using bone in chicken, remove the bones and return chicken to pot.
5. Stir in the olives and raisins and serve hot on top of rice

Prep: 10 mins

Cook: 30

Total: 40 mins

Servings: 5

Ingredients

- 1 lb ground breakfast sausage
- 12 oz extra firm tofu pressed
- 1 medium sweet potato ½ inch dice
- 1 yellow onion diced
- 2 small carrots shredded
- 1 cup loose packed spinach coarse chop
- 3 cups cooked brown rice
- 2 cloves garlic minced
- 1 tsp dried rosemary
- 2 tsp salt or to taste
- ½ tsp black pepper
- 1 tbsp nutritional yeast

- ¼ tsp turmeric
- 2 tsp soy sauce

Directions

1. Brown the ground sausage over medium low heat in a large skillet.
2. Remove browned sausage and set aside.
3. Add the onion and carrots to the sauage greased pan and saute for about 6-8 minutes stirring occasionally, until onions are translucent, carrots may stick a bit.
4. Add the sweet potato to the pan and stir, leave undisturbed for 5-7 minutes, you want the potatoes to brown a bit.
5. Stir, add a splash of water, cover pan and cook for 10 more minutes.
6. Add the garlic and rosemary and saute a minute longer.
7. Scrape veggies to one side of the pan and add the tofu to the empty side.

8. Break up the tofu in the pan so that it is in small pieces.

9. Add the salt, pepper, nutritional yeast, turmeric, and soy sauce to the tofu and mix.

10. Stir the entire contents of the pan together.

11. Add the spinach and heat just until it starts to wilt, about 3 minutes.

12. Stir in the sausage and serve warm over rice.

Prep: 20 mins

Cook: 30 mins

Total: 50 mins

Servings: 5

Ingredients

- 2-3 lb pork tenderloin, trimmed
- 1 15 oz can peaches in juice, not syrup
- 1 stalk celery, sliced thin
- 2 medium yellow onions, sliced thin
- 1 bay leaf
- 2 tsp rosemary
- 1 tsp salt
- 1/2 tsp black pepper
- 1/2 cup chicken broth
- olive oil

Directions

1. Preheat oven to 400 degrees F.
2. Heat an oven safe skillet or dutch oven over medium high heat, drizzle with olive oil.
3. Brown pork tenderloin on all sides, 1-2 minutes a side.
4. Set pork tenderloin aside.
5. Reduce heat to medium low, add onion and celery to the pan and saute for 10-12 minutes, until the onions take on the brown of the pork drippings.
6. Add the can of peaches complete with juice, scrape off any pork bits on the bottom.
7. Add the remaining ingredients and return the pork to the pan.
8. Move the pan to the oven and cook for 25-30 minutes until internal temperature reaches 145 degrees F.
9. Serve warm with your favorite sides.

Prep: 15 mins

Cook: 1 hr

Total: 1 hr 15 mins

Servings: 4

Ingredients

- 1 large sweet potato, peeled and diced
- ½ medium zucchini, shredded
- ½ medium yellow squash, shredded
- 1 pound ground turkey
- black pepper to taste

Directions

1. Place sweet potatoes into a large pot and cover with salted water; bring to a boil. Reduce heat to medium-low and simmer until tender, about 20

minutes. Drain. Mash sweet potatoes with a fork in a large bowl; set aside to cool.

2. Preheat the oven to 350 degrees F (175 degrees C).

3. Mix zucchini and yellow squash into the bowl with the sweet potatoes. Add turkey and black pepper. Form mixture into 1-inch balls and place in a 9x13-inch baking dish.

4. Bake in the preheated oven until meatballs are no longer pink in the center, 35 to 40 minutes.

Prep: 15 mins

Cook: 1 hr

Total: 1 hr 15 mins

Servings: 12

Ingredients

Dry:

- 2 cups finely ground oat flour
- ½ tsp baking soda, remove for high altitude
- 1 tsp baking powder
- 1 tsp ground cinnamon
- ¼ tsp salt

Wet:

- ⅓ cup melted coconut oil
- ¼ cup sugar
- ¼ real maple syrup

- 1 ½ flax eggs 4 ½ tsp ground flaxseed whisked into ¼ cup water, let sit for 15 mins
- 1 tsp vanilla extract

Fold- ins:

- 1 ¼ cup grated zucchini
- ½ cup raisins

Directions

1. Preheat the oven to 325 degrees F.
2. Line a 8 inch loaf pan with parchment paper, or grease all sides with coconut oil
3. In a medium bowl mix the dry ingredients.
4. In a larger bowl combine all wet ingredients.
5. Add the dry ingredients to the wet ingredients, mixing as you add.
6. Make sure dry ingredients are fully incorporated and then fold in zucchini and raisins.
7. Pour the thick batter into the lined pan and shape into a loaf.

8. Bake for 60-70 minutes, until internal temp reaches 200 degrees F, the loaf will look pale.

9. Cool the loaf in the pan for at least half an hour before removing, allow it to cool completely before serving.

Prep: 40 mins

Cook: 1 hr

Total: 1 hr 40 mins

Servings: 10

Ingredients

- 250g dried garbanzo beans (or 2 cans)
- 1⁄2 cup sunflower oil
- 3⁄4 cup water, retain from cooking
- 1⁄3 cup tahini
- 3⁄4 teaspoon salt
- 1 garlic clove

Optional batch of Spinach Hummus

- 5 ounces frozen spinach (optional)
- 1 1⁄2 teaspoons dried parsley (optional)

Directions

1. Night before- If using dried peas bring the peas to a boil in 5 cups of water. Boil for three minutes, then remove from heat and cover. Leave overnight.
2. Drain and rinse the peas (both dried & canned) in batches and place on a paper towel. Run each batch over with a rolling pin. Then remove any loose skins.
3. Once the skins are removed, place in pressure cooker with 5 cups of water. Bring to pressure and cook for 25 minutes and let pressure drop naturally.
4. Drain the chickpeas, but make sure to retain a 1/2 cup of cooking water.
5. Pour all the chickpeas in the food processor and add all the other ingredients. You want to blend them for about 2 minutes. The longer you blend it the smoother it is. It goes very creamy when you've got it right.
6. The mixture will be a bit runny, it firms up as it cools.

7. Optional: Remove about half the hummus (500-600 grams) and add the spinach and parsley. Blend again until even.

Prep: 5 mins

Servings: 1

Ingredients

- 1/2 cup rolled oats
- 1 cup coconut milk or plain or vanilla milk of choice
- 1/2 cup pitted cherries fresh or frozen
- splash vanilla extract
- dash salt
- 1 tbsp unsweetened cocoa powder
- 1/4 tsp cinnamon
- 1 tbsp sweetened shredded coconut optional

Directions

- Place oats, milk, cherries, vanilla, cocoa, and salt in a microwave safe bowl.
- Microwave for 90 seconds.

- Remove and stir.

- Microwave for another 90 seconds for frozen cherries, 30 seconds for fresh.

- Stir again and let sit for 2-5 minutes.

- Top with cinnamon and shredded coconut and enjoy hot.

Prep: 5 mins

Cook: 15 mins

Total: 20 mins

Servings: 2

Ingredients

- 2 zucchini, sliced thinly
- 2 carrots, sliced thinly
- 2 tsp avocado oil or ghee
- 4 tsp water
- 2 boneless, skinless salmon filets less than 1 1/4" thick
- 1 clove garlic diced
- sea salt and black pepper to taste

Directions

1. Preheat oven to 450 degrees F. Toss vegetables with olive oil.

2. Tear two sheets of parchment paper and fold in half. Open the sheets and place half of the vegetables onto each sheet on one side of the fold. Add 2 teaspoons of water and place a fillet on top. Top with garlic, salt, and pepper.

3. Fold the other half of each sheet over the fish, and tightly crimp the edges. Put packets flat on a baking sheet and bake for 10-15 minutes.

4. Remove from oven and check to ensure fish flakes easily with a fork (be careful the steam is hot). Open each pack and place onto plates. Serve & enjoy!

Prep: 5 mins

Cook: 25 mins

Total: 30 mins

Servings: 6

Ingredients

- 400 g cubed frozen butternut squash (roughly 2.5 cups)
- 2 tbsp garlic infused olive oil
- 1 cup oat milk (or other dairy free milk of choice)
- 4 tbsp nutritional yeast
- 1/2 tsp salt
- 150 g gluten-free macaroni (roughly 1.5 cups)

Directions

1. Heat your pan to medium heat and add 2 tablespoons of garlic infused olive oil.

2. Add frozen butternut squash cubes.

3. Cook until butternut squash is fully thawed and cooked through, stirring often.

4. While your butternut squash is cooking, bring a large pot of water to a boil. Salt the water generously and add your gluten-free pasta, stirring often until cooked through. Follow the instructions on the packaging and be careful not to overcook.

5. Add oat milk, nutritional yeast and ½ teaspoon salt to your butternut squash.

6. Continue cooking until all the flavors have started combining, around five minutes. Stir often. Turn the heat off and let the butternut squash mixture cool down a bit.

7. At this point your pasta will likely be done. Strain your pasta and set aside.

8. Once your butternut squash mixture has cooled a bit, transfer it into a food processor or blender and blend until smooth.

9. Add your sauce to your cooked pasta and stir everything together.

10. Serve immediately.

Prep: 1 hr 10 mins

Cook: 30 mins

Total: 1 hr 40 mins

Servings: 5

Ingredients

For the Chicken:

- 5 boneless chicken thighs
- 3 cups cooked jasmine or basmati rice
- 16 oz can of pineapple chunks drained
- 2 medium yellow onions
- 2 large carrots sliced
- olive oil
- salt and pepper

For the Sauce:

- 1 tbsp arrowroot powder
- 1 tbsp cold water

- ½ cup brown sugar
- ½ cup coconut aminos
- ¼ cup apple cider vinegar
- 1 tsp ground ginger
- ¼ tsp black pepper

Directions

1. Lightly oil a 9×9 baking dish.
2. Place chicken thighs in baking dish.
3. Whisk together the sauce ingredients minus the arrowroot powder, make sure it's well combined.
4. Whisk the arrowroot powder into the sauce.
5. Pour sauce over the chicken thighs.
6. Add sliced carrots on top of the chicken.
7. Refrigerate to marinate for at least 1 hour.
8. Preheat oven to 400 degrees F.
9. Bake chicken for 30 minutes until internal temp reaches 160 degrees F.
10. While chicken is baking, heat olive oil in medium pan over medium low heat.

11. Add sliced onions and caramelize slowly, you want to really bring the sugars out and are looking for a dark brown color.

12. When the onions have reached peak caramel add fully drained pineapple chunks and season with salt and pepper to taste.

13. Bring a brown to the pineapple and then add the cooked rice to the pan.

14. Remove chicken from oven and pour extra sauce into pan with rice, toss well.

15. Serve with the chicken thighs topping the rice mixture.

Prep: 5 mins

Cook: 20 mins

Total: 25 mins

Servings: 4

Ingredients

- ½ cup rice flour
- ½ cup coconut or oat milk, plain or vanilla is fine
- 1 ripe banana, peeled
- pinch salt
- coconut oil
- real maple syrup for serving

Directions

1. In a blender or food processor combine all ingredients except coconut oil and maple syrup.
2. Blend for about 30 seconds until very smooth.

3. Heat a skillet over medium low heat, grease with coconut oil.

4. Pour batter into pancake rounds on heated skillet, how many depends on the size of your skillet.

5. Cook for about 4 minutes before flipping and cooking for another 3 minutes, both sides should be a deep golden brown, keep the heat at medium low to get it cooked all the way through without burning.

6. Repeat until batter is used up, re-grease the pan as needed.

7. Serve hot with real maple syrup or favorite pancake topping.

Prep: 15 mins

Cook: 20 mins

Total: 35 mins

Servings: 6

Ingredients

- 3 cups shredded chicken
- 3 cups cooked brown rice
- 1 medium onion, chopped
- 2 medium carrots, shredded
- 4 cups small broccoli florets
- 1 tbsp brown mustard
- 1 tsp dried parsley
- ½ tsp dried thyme
- ¾ tsp salt
- ¼ tsp pepper
- ½ cup chicken broth
- 1 batch vegan, nut free, alfredo sauce

- ½ batch vegan, nut free, parmesan topping
- olive oil

Directions

1. Preheat oven to 350 degrees F
2. Heat a skillet over medium low, drizzle with olive oil.
3. Saute the onion and carrot for 7-10 minutes until onions turn clear.
4. Add the broccoli and heat just until the florets turn bright green, about 2-3 minutes.
5. In a large mixing bowl, combine sauteed vegetables, chicken, rice, and vegan, nut free, alfredo sauce.
6. In a small bowl, whisk together chicken broth and mustard, parsley, thyme, salt, and pepper.
7. Place the chicken mixture in a greased 9×13 casserole dish.
8. Pour chicken broth mixture even over the casserole.
9. Top with vegan, nut free, parmesean topping.

10. Bake for 20 minutes to heat all the way through.

11. Serve hot!

Prep: 10 mins

Cook: 25mins

Total: 35 mins

Servings: 6

Ingredients

- 1-2 tbsp canola oil
- 1/2 cup celery, chopped
- 1/2 cup carrots, chopped
- 1/2 cup leeks
- 1/2 tsp (1 clove) garlic, minced
- 1 large or 2 medium russet potatoes, peeled and cut into 1" pieces (about 2 cups)
- 4-5 cups water or FAILSAFE broth
- 1 (15 oz) can black beans, drained and rinsed
- 3/4 cup dried green lentils
- 1 tsp salt (or more to taste)

Directions

1. Heat 1 tbsp canola oil in a large stock pot over medium heat. Add in celery, leeks, and carrots (if you can tolerate) and sauté for about 3-5 minutes or until vegetables become bright and fragrant.
2. Add in garlic and sauté for another minute more.
3. Add in potatoes and continue to cook for another 3-5 minutes.
4. Add in broth, black beans, and lentils and bring to a boil.
5. Reduce heat to low and simmer for 25 minutes or until potatoes are fork tender and lentils are done cooking. Adjust salt to taste.

Prep: 10 mins

Cook: 1 hr

Total: 1 hr 10 mins

Servings: 5

Ingredients

For the Stir Fry:

- 5 bone in chicken thighs
- 1 large carrot, halved lengthwise and sliced
- 1 yellow onion diced
- 3 stalks bok choy white parts only, halved lengthwise and sliced
- 8 ounces of your favorite mushroom, sliced
- ¼ head of cabbage about 2 cups, chopped
- salt pepper, and olive oil
- 4 cups cooked brown basmatti, or jasmine rice

For the Sauce:

- ¼ cup coconut milk full fat preferred
- ¼ real maple syrup, no corn syrup.
- 2 tsp fresh grated ginger; powdered okay just lower to 1 tsp
- ½ tsp turmeric
- splash of rice vinegar
- 1 tsp salt or to taste

Directions

1. Preheat oven to 450 degrees F.
2. Heat cast iron skillet on stove top at medium low, just make sure the pan is hot!
3. Rub olive oil onto skins of chicken thighs and liberally season with salt and pepper.
4. Place chicken thighs skin side down in heated cast iron (it should sizzle!)
5. Cook the thighs skin side down for about 7-10 minutes until the skin is golden brown and crispy.

6. Flip thighs over and place whole skillet into the oven for 20-25 minutes until the thighs reach an internal temp of 165 degrees F.
7. While the thighs are cooking, whisk together sauce ingredients (using a fork works too!)
8. Remove thighs from oven, place thighs skin up on a paper towel lined plate to rest.
9. Return cast iron to stovetop at medium heat, leave all the fat in! (if you really want to, you can drain half of it but more fat is more flavor).
10. Stir fry the chopped veggies in all the chicken fat for about 15-20 minutes until they reach the desired texture and the mushrooms sweat their liquid completely.
11. Remove the thigh meat from the bones and toss with the veggies and sauce off of the heat.
12. Serve on rice.

Prep: 20 mins

Cook: 30 mins

Total: 50 mins

Servings: 5

Ingredients

- 1 1/2 pounds lean ground beef
- 1 tbsp ground flaxseed
- 3 tbsp cool water
- 1/8 cup rolled oats
- 1/4 cup oat milk
- 1 tbsp coconut aminos or soy sauce
- 1 tsp fish sauce
- 2 tsp brown mustard
- 1/2 tsp onion powder
- 1/2 tsp garlic powder
- 1/2 tsp oregano
- 1 tsp dried parsley

- 1 tsp salt
- 1/2 tsp black pepper
- 6 tbsp cherry ketchup

Directions

1. Preheat oven to 350 degrees F.
2. Combine the ground flaxseed in cool water in a medium mixing bowl and set aside for 10-15 minutes.
3. Add the remaining ingredients except the cherrry ketchup to the bowl and thoroughly mix.
4. Grease a muffin tin, about 10 cups.
5. Press the beef mixture into the greased muffin cups.
6. Place the muffin tin on a larger baking tray just in case any grease drips.
7. Bake mini meat loaves for 20 minutes.
8. Remove from the oven and top each mini meatloaf with cherry ketchup.
9. Return to oven for 5-10 minutes until internal temperature reaches 160 degrees F and serve hot.

Prep: 15 mins

Cook: 15mins

Total: 30 mins

Servings: 8

Ingredients

For the poached chicken:

- 2 lb chicken
- 2 smashed garlic clove
- 2 tablespoon fresh oregano, roughly chopped
- 1/2 of an onion, roughly chopped
- 1 teaspoon salt
- 6 cup water, or enough to cover the chicken

For the soup:

- 4 teaspoon canola oil
- 4 carrots, diced small
- Half onion, diced

- 4 garlic cloves, minced
- 12 cup broth (can use the strained poaching liquid from the chicken)
- 1 1/2 cup uncooked quinoa
- 4 cup poached chicken
- 2 handful of fresh baby kale
- 2 teaspoon salt
- ½ teaspoon black pepper
- ½ cup fresh dill, chopped

Directions

1. To poach the chicken, place all of the ingredients for the poached chicken in a medium sized pot. Cover and bring the water to a boil, keep covered and reduce heat to low simmering for 10-14 minutes. The internal temperature of the chicken should be 165 °F. Shred the chicken with forks once cooked.
2. For the soup, heat a large soup pot over medium heat and add the canola oil. Once heated, add the

carrots, onion, and garlic. Cook, stirring frequently until soft, about 5 minutes.

3. Add the broth and the quinoa. Bring to a boil, then cover and reduce the heat to low. Cook the quinoa for about 10 minutes.

4. Once the quinoa is soft, add the poached chicken, baby kale, salt, pepper, and fresh dill.

27. Brunch Baked Sweet Potatoes

Prep: 20 mins

Cook: 1 hr

Total: 1 hr 20 mins

Servings: 4

Ingredients

- 4 medium sweet potatoes
- 1 lb ground breakfast sausage no corn syrup or nightshades
- 1/2 red onion thinly sliced
- 1/4 cup white vinegar
- 2 tbsp sugar
- 1/2 tsp salt
- 1/2 tsp black pepper
- 2 cups mixed greens
- 2 ripe avocados sliced
- 2 tsp salted roasted, sunflower seeds
- 4 tbsp real maple syrup

- additional salt and pepper to taste

Directions

1. Preheat oven to 400 degrees F.
2. Wrap whole sweet potatoes in aluminum foil.
3. Bake for 45-60 minutes, until softened through.
4. While the potatoes are baking, brown the sausage, drain and set aside.
5. Also while baking combine the vinegar, sugar, salt, and pepper in a small sauce pan and bring to a boil.
6. Remove vinegar mixture from heat and add the sliced red onions, stir well and set aside.
7. When the potatoes have been cooked remove from foil and place on 4 plates.
8. Cut the potatoes lengthwise, top with browned sausage and all remaining ingredients portioned into 4.
9. Drizzle with the maple syrup last and sprinkle with salt and pepper. Then serve warm.

Prep: 20 mins

Cook: 1 hr

Total: 1 hr 20 mins

Servings: 4

Ingredients

For the crust:

- 1 large sweet potato
- 1 tsp salt
- 1 tsp garlic powder
- 2 tsp onion powder
- ⅓ cup oat flour (can be homemade slightly coarse)
- 2 eggs
- coconut or olive oil

For the Filling:

- ½ small head of broccoli small florets
- ½ small head of cauliflower small florets

- ⅓ lb of ham cubes about 1 cm in width
- 8 green onions white parts included, chopped
- 3 eggs
- ⅔ cup oat milk or prefered plain milk
- salt and pepper

Directions

For the Crust:

1. Preheat oven to 325 degrees F.
2. Grease a 9 inch pie dish (not loose bottom) with coconut or olive oil.
3. Grate the potato and squeeze out excess moisture using a tea towel.
4. Mix potato, seasonings, and oat flour in a medium bowl.
5. Add one egg and mix until incorporated.
6. Press the mixture into the greased dish along the bottom and up the sides.
7. Brush the crust with half of the other egg, all along the bottom and sides.
8. Bake crust for 25-30 minutes.

9. Remove the crust and brush again with the remaining egg, fill any gaps!

10. Bake crust for another 5 minutes.

For the Quiche:

1. Put the vegetables and ham into the prebaked crust, make sure it's an even mix and the ingredients aren't segregated.

2. Whisk the egg and milk together in a small bowl.

3. Pour egg mixture over the top of the ham and veggies, try to fill in every little space.

4. Sprinkle top with salt and pepper (however much you prefer).

5. Bake for 25-35 minutes until crust edges are deep brown, if you like your egg softer lean toward the 25 minute side.

6. Remove from oven and cool for 30 minutes before serving.

Prep: 20 mins

Cook: 55 mins

Total: 1 hr 15 mins

Servings: 4

Ingredients

- 1 13.5 oz Can of canned coconut milk
- 3 medium ripe bananas
- 1 10 oz bag of shredded carrots
- 3/4 cup unsweetened shredded coconut
- 1/4 cup coconut flour
- 2 tbsp pure maple syrup
- 1/2 tsp baking soda
- 2 tsp cinnamon
- 1 tsp nutmeg
- 1/2 tsp all spice optional

Directions

1. Preheat oven to 350 degrees.
2. In a large mixing bowl, combine all ingredients until evenly mixed.
3. Scoop the mixture into a glass 9×13 dish.
4. Pat with hand or spatula to ensure the mixture is even.
5. Cover pan with foil and bake for about 55 minutes or until the n'oatmeal is moist.
6. Let cool for 5-7 minutes then scoop out and enjoy!
7. Top with your favorite toppings such as more shredded coconut or raw cacao nibs.

Prep: 15 mins

Cook: 30 mins

Total: 45 mins

Servings: 4

Ingredients

- 2 tablespoons extra-virgin olive oil
- 1 teaspoon chili powder
- 1 teaspoon garlic powder
- ½ teaspoon ground cumin
- ¼ teaspoon salt
- 1 pound flank steak, trimmed
- 4 cups sliced onions
- 2 cups sliced bell peppers
- 2 cups sliced poblano peppers
- 8 (6 inch) corn tortillas, warmed
- ½ cup guacamole
- Lime wedges for serving

- Cilantro for garnish

Directions

1. Position racks in upper and lower thirds of oven and place a large rimmed baking sheet on each; preheat to 500 degrees F.

2. Combine oil, chili powder, garlic powder, cumin and salt in a large bowl. Rub steak with half of the spice mixture. Add onions, bell peppers and poblanos to the bowl and toss to coat.

3. Carefully place the steak on the pan on the top rack and carefully spread the vegetables on the pan on the lower rack. Roast until the steak and vegetables are starting to brown, about 8 minutes.

4. Flip the steak and stir the vegetables. Turn the broiler to high and continue cooking the steak to desired doneness (an instant-read thermometer inserted in the thickest part will register 120 degrees F for medium rare) and the vegetables until charred, about 6 minutes more. Transfer the steak to a cutting board and let rest for 5 minutes.

5. Slice the steak across the grain and serve in tortillas with the vegetables and guacamole. Serve with lime wedges and cilantro, if desired.